Quick And Easy Comfort Food Recipe Collection For Busy People

Effortless and affordable comfort food cooking guide

Jane Ball

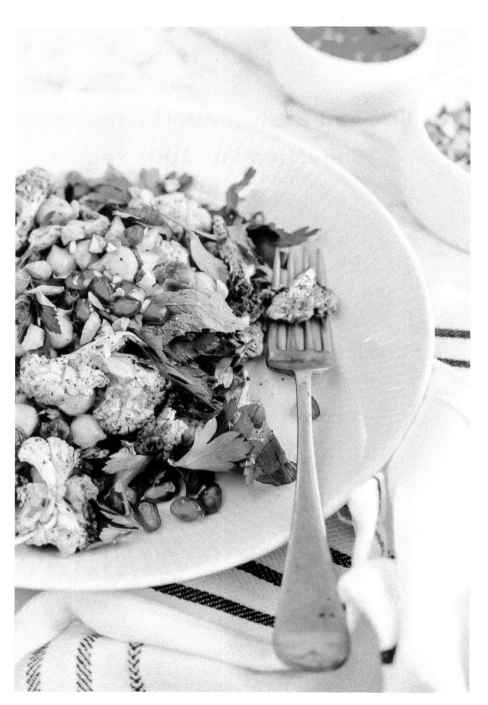

professional advice. The content within this book has been derived from various sources. Please consult a licensed professional before attempting any techniques outlined in this book.

By reading this document, the reader agrees that under no circumstances is the author responsible for any losses, direct or indirect, which are incurred as a result of the use of information contained within this document, including, but not limited to, — errors, omissions, or inaccuracies.

Table of contents

Goat Cheese Cauliflower

Preparation time: 25 minutes | Cooking Time: 15 minutes | Servings: 4

Ingredients:

8 cups cauliflower florets; roughly chopped.

4 bacon strips; chopped.

10 oz. Goat cheese, crumbled

¼ cup soft cream cheese

½ cup spring onions; chopped.

1 tbsp. Garlic; minced

Salt and black pepper to taste.

Cooking spray

Directions:

Grease a baking pan that fits the air fryer with the cooking spray and mix all the ingredients except the goat cheese into the pan.

Sprinkle the cheese on top, introduce the pan in the machine and cook at 400°F for 20 minutes

Divide between plates and serve as a side dish.

Nutrition:

Calories 203, Fat 13g, Fiber 2g, Carbs 5g, Protein 9g.

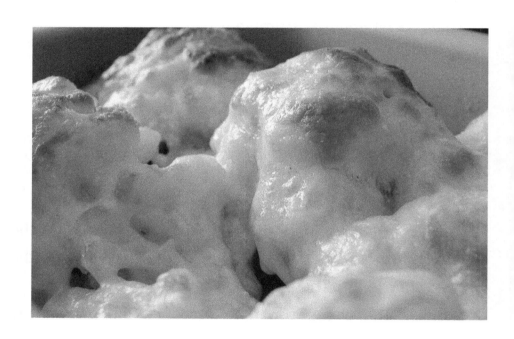

Dill Red Cabbage

Preparation time: 25 minutes | Cooking Time: 15 minutes | Servings: 4

Ingredients:

30 oz. Red cabbage; shredded

4 oz. Butter; melted

1 tbsp. Red wine vinegar

2 tbsp. Dill; chopped.

1 tsp. Cinnamon powder

A pinch of salt and black pepper

Directions:

In a pan that fits your air fryer, mix the cabbage with the rest of the ingredients, toss put the pan in the machine, and cook at 390°F for 20 minutes

Divide between plates and serve as a side dish.

Nutrition:

Calories 201, Fat 17g, Fiber 2g, Carbs 5g, Protein 5g.

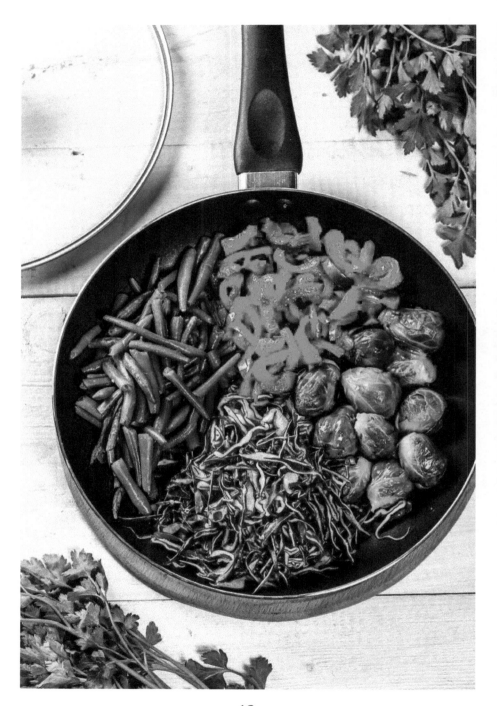

Radishes and Sesame Seeds

Preparation time: 20 minutes | Cooking Time: 15 minutes | Servings: 4

Ingredients:

20 radishes; halved

2 spring onions; chopped.

3 green onions; chopped.

2 tbsp. Olive oil

1 tbsp. Olive oil

3 tsp. Black sesame seeds

Salt and black pepper to taste.

Directions:

Take a bowl and mix all the ingredients and toss well.

Put the radishes in your air fryer's basket, cook at 400°F for 15 minutes, divide between plates and serve as a side dish

Nutrition:

Calories 150, Fat 4g, Fiber 2g, Carbs 3g, Protein 5g.

220. Herbed Radish Sauté

Preparation time: 20 minutes | Cooking Time: 15 minutes | Servings: 4

Ingredients:

2 bunches red radishes; halved

2 tbsp. Parsley; chopped.

2 tbsp. Balsamic vinegar

1 tbsp. Olive oil

Salt and black pepper to taste.

Directions:

Take a bowl and mix the radishes with the remaining ingredients except the parsley, toss and put them in your air fryer's basket.

Cook at 400°F for 15 minutes, divide between plates, sprinkle the parsley on top and serve as a side dish

Nutrition:

Calories 180, Fat 4g, Fiber 2g, Carbs 3g, Protein 5g.

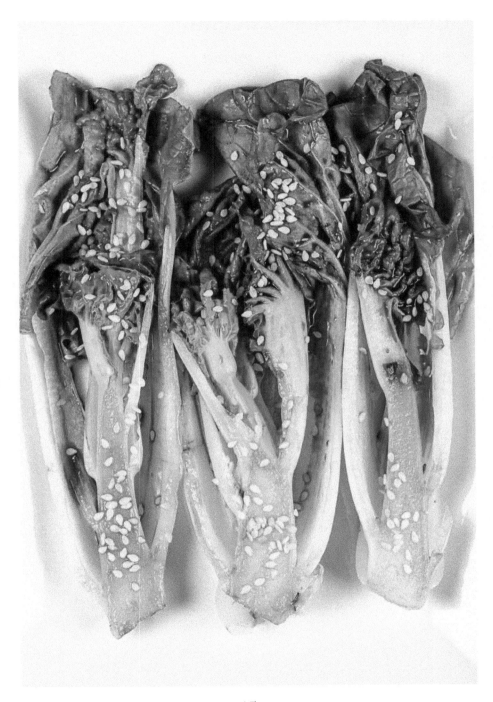

Cream Cheese Zucchini

Preparation time: 20 minutes | Cooking Time: 15 minutes | Servings: 4

Ingredients:

1 lb. Zucchinis; cut into wedges

1 green onion; sliced

1 cup cream cheese, soft

1 tbsp. Butter; melted

2 tbsp. Basil; chopped.

1 tsp. Garlic powder

A pinch of salt and black pepper

Directions:

In a pan that fits your air fryer, mix the zucchinis with all the other ingredients, toss, introduce in the air fryer and cook at 370°F for 15 minutes

Divide between plates and serve as a side dish.

Nutrition:

Calories 129, Fat 6g, Fiber 2g, Carbs 5g, Protein 8g.

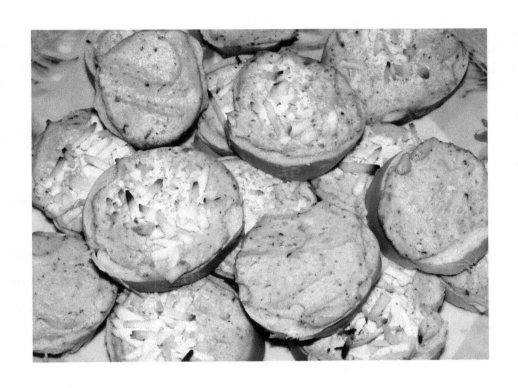

Sausage Mushroom Caps

Preparation time: 18 minutes | Cooking Time: 15 minutes | Servings: 2

Ingredients:

½ lb. Italian sausage

6 large portobello mushroom caps

¼ cup grated parmesan cheese.

¼ cup chopped onion

2 tbsp. Blanched finely ground almond flour

1 tsp. Minced fresh garlic

Directions:

Use a spoon to hollow out each mushroom cap, reserving scrapings.

In a medium skillet over medium heat, brown the sausage about 10 minutes or until fully cooked and no pink remains. Drain and then add reserved mushroom scrapings, onion, almond flour, parmesan, and garlic.

Gently fold ingredients together and continue cooking an additional minute, then remove from heat

Evenly spoon the mixture into mushroom caps and place the caps into a 6-inch round pan. Place pan into the air fryer basket

Adjust the temperature to 375° F and set the timer for 8 minutes. When finished cooking, the tops will be browned and bubbling. Serve warm.

Nutrition:

Calories 404, Protein 24.3g, Fiber 4.5g, Fat 25.8g, Carbs 18.2g.

Minty Summer Squash

Preparation time: 30 minutes | Cooking Time: 15 minutes | Servings: 4

Ingredients:

4 summer squash; cut into wedges

½ cup mint; chopped.

1 cup mozzarella; shredded

¼ cup olive oil

¼ cup lemon juice

Salt and black pepper to taste.

Directions:

In a pan that fits your air fryer, mix the squash with the rest of the ingredients, toss, introduce the pan in the air fryer and cook at 370°F for 25 minutes

Divide between plates and serve as a side dish.

Nutrition:

Calories 201, Fat 7g, Fiber 2g, Carbs 4g, Protein 9g.

Air Fried Ratatouille

Preparation Time: 10 minutes | Cooking Time: 15 minutes | Servings: 6

Ingredients:

1 eggplant, diced

2 bell peppers, diced

1 tbsp vinegar

1 1/2 tbsp olive oil

2 tbsp herb de Provence

3 garlic cloves, chopped

1 onion, diced

3 tomatoes, diced

Pepper

Salt

Directions:

Line Pressure Pot multi-level air fryer basket with foil.

Add all ingredients into the bowl and toss well and transfer into the air fryer basket and place the basket into the Pressure Pot.

Seal pot with air fryer lid and select air fry mode then set the temperature to 400° F and timer for 15 minutes. Stir halfway through.

Serve and enjoy.

Nutrition:

Calories 91, Fat 4.3g, Carbohydrates 12.1g, Sugar 6.7g, Protein 2.9g, Cholesterol 0mg.

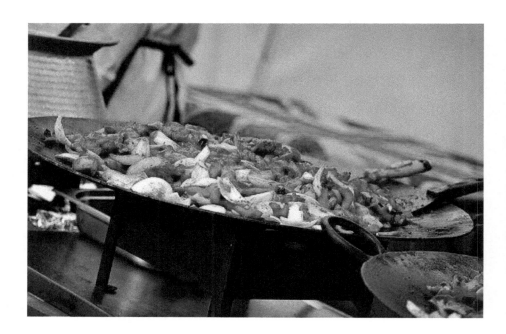

Squash Casserole

Preparation Time: 10 minutes | Cooking Time: 35 minutes | Servings: 8

Ingredients:

4 1/2 lbs yellow squash, cut into bite-size pieces

2 tbsp mayonnaise

1 1/2 cups cheddar cheese, shredded

1 egg, lightly beaten

10 oz cream of celery soup

1 cup onion, chopped

Pepper

Salt

For topping:

1/2 cup butter, melted

1 cup crushed crackers

Directions:

Add squash pieces into the boiling water and boil until tender. Drain well and set aside.

Mix squash, onion, celery soup, egg, mayonnaise, pepper, and salt and pour into the Pressure Pot.

Sprinkle cheddar cheese on top.

Seal pot with air fryer lid and select bake mode then set the temperature to 350° F and timer for 20 minutes.

Mix butter and crushed crackers and sprinkle on top. Seal pot with air fryer lid and select bake mode then set the temperature to 350° F and timer for 15 minutes. Serve and enjoy.

Nutrition:

Calories 281, Fat 22.4g, Carbohydrates 13.6g, Sugar 5.9g, Protein 9.8g, Cholesterol 78mg.

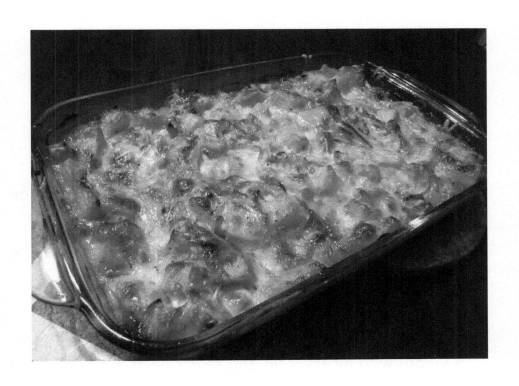

Corn Gratin

Preparation Time: 10 minutes | Cooking Time: 30 minutes | Servings: 8

Ingredients:

2 cups corn

1 cup cheddar cheese, shredded

1 cup milk

1 tbsp flour

1 tbsp butter

1 cup crushed crackers

Directions:

Add butter into the Pressure Pot and set the pot on sauté mode.

Add flour and milk and stir until smooth. Turn off the sauté mode.

Add corn and cup cheese and stir well.

Sprinkle remaining cheese and crushed crackers on top.

Seal pot with air fryer lid and select bake mode then set the temperature to 350° F and timer for 15 minutes.

Serve and enjoy.

Nutrition:

Calories 137, Fat 8g, Carbohydrates 11.6g, Sugar 3.1g, Protein 6.1g, Cholesterol 21mg.

Flavors Crab Casserole

Preparation Time: 10 minutes | Cooking Time: 30 minutes | Servings: 5

Ingredients:

8 oz crabmeat

1 onion, sliced

1/4 tsp garlic powder

1/4 tsp onion powder

1 tsp Worcestershire sauce

1 cup Swiss cheese, shredded

1 cup cheddar cheese, shredded

1/4 cup sour cream

5 oz cream cheese

Directions:

Spray Pressure Pot from inside with cooking spray.

Add all ingredients except cheddar cheese into the Pressure Pot and stir well.

Sprinkle cheddar cheese on top.

Seal pot with air fryer lid and select bake mode then set the temperature to 350° F and timer for 30 minutes.

Serve and enjoy.

Nutrition:

Calories 350, Fat 26g, Carbohydrates 11.9g, Sugar 4.5g, Protein 17.7g, Cholesterol 89mg.

Broccoli Chicken Casserole

Preparation Time: 10 minutes | Cooking Time: 25 minutes | Servings: 6

Ingredients:

3 chicken breasts, boneless, cooked and diced

1/2 cup breadcrumbs

1 cup cheddar cheese, shredded

2 tbsp parmesan cheese, grated

1 tsp lemon juice

3/4 cup milk

10 oz broccoli florets, cooked and drained

10 oz cream of chicken soup

Directions:

Spray Pressure Pot from inside with cooking spray.

Add chicken, lemon juice, milk, broccoli, and soup into the Pressure Pot and stir well.

Sprinkle cheddar cheese, parmesan cheese, and breadcrumbs on top.

Seal pot with air fryer lid and select bake mode then set the temperature to 350° F and timer for 25 minutes.

Serve and enjoy.

Nutrition:

Calories 330, Fat 16.1g, Carbohydrates 14.8g, Sugar 3.1g, Protein 31.1g, Cholesterol 92mg.

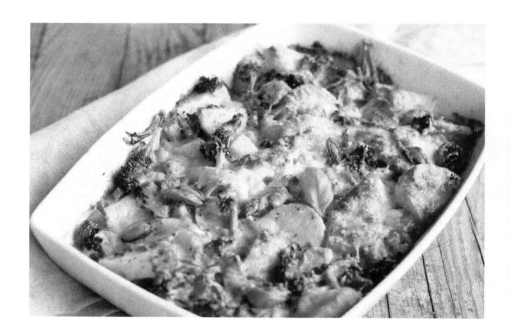

Cauliflower Casserole

Preparation Time: 10 minutes | Cooking Time: 25 minutes | Servings: 6

Ingredients:

1 cauliflower head, cut into florets

1 1/2 cups cheddar cheese, shredded

3/4 cup heavy cream

Pepper

Salt

Directions:

Spray Pressure Pot from inside with cooking spray.

Add cauliflower florets into the boiling water and cook for 6 minutes. Drain well.

Add cauliflower florets, 1/2 cup cheddar cheese, heavy cream, pepper, and salt into the Pressure Pot and stir well.

Sprinkle remaining cheddar cheese on top.

Seal pot with air fryer lid and select bake mode then set the temperature to 350° F and timer for 20 minutes.

Serve and enjoy.

Nutrition:

Calories 177, Fat 15g, Carbohydrates 3.1g, Sugar 1.2g, Protein 8.2g Cholesterol 50mg.

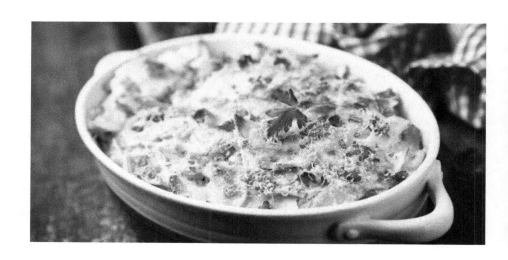

Buffalo Chicken Casserole

Preparation Time: 10 minutes | Cooking Time: 30 minutes | Servings: 8

Ingredients:

18 oz cauliflower florets

1 cup celery, chopped

12 oz chicken, cooked and diced

8 oz cheddar cheese, shredded

2 eggs, lightly beaten

1/4 cup ranch dressing

1/3 cup hot sauce

8 oz cream cheese

Directions:

Spray Pressure Pot from inside with cooking spray.

Add cauliflower florets into the boiling water and cook for 6 minutes. Drain well and set aside.

Add cauliflower florets, chicken, and celery into the Pressure Pot.

In a bowl, mix cream cheese, hot sauce, ranch dressing, eggs, and 4 oz cheddar cheese and pour over cauliflower mixture.

Sprinkle remaining cheddar cheese on top.

Seal pot with air fryer lid and select bake mode then set the temperature to 350° F and timer for 30 minutes. Serve and enjoy.

Nutrition:

Calories 314, Fat 21.8g, Carbohydrates 5.5g, Sugar 2.3g, Protein 24.4g, Cholesterol 135mg.

Turkey Stroganoff

Preparation Time: 10 minutes | Cooking Time: 34 minutes | Servings: 8

Ingredients:

12 oz egg noodles, cooked and drained

1/4 cup parmesan cheese, grated

2 cups cooked turkey, diced

1 cup sour cream

2 cups chicken broth

1/4 cup all-purpose flour

1 tbsp parsley, chopped

8 oz mushrooms, sliced

2 tbsp butter

Directions:

Add butter into the Pressure Pot and set the pot on sauté mode.

Add mushrooms and sauté for 3-4 minutes. remove mushrooms from the pot and set them aside.

Add flour, sour cream, and broth and stir until smooth. Turn off the sauté mode.

Add noodles, turkey, mushrooms, and parsley and stir well.

Sprinkle parmesan cheese on top.

Seal pot with air fryer lid and select bake mode then set the temperature to 350° F and timer for 30 minutes. Serve and enjoy.

Nutrition:

Calories 244, Fat 12.6g, Carbohydrates 16.2g, Sugar 0.9g, Protein 16.5g, Cholesterol 61mg.

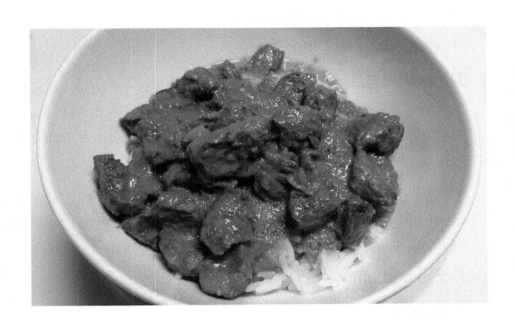

Turkey Casserole

Preparation Time: 10 minutes | Cooking Time: 40 minutes | Servings: 8

Ingredients:

6 cups cooked turkey, shredded

1 cup milk

2 cans cream of chicken soup

4 cups bread stuffing

Directions:

Spray Pressure Pot from inside with cooking spray.

Add milk, soup, and turkey into the Pressure Pot and stir well.

Sprinkle bread stuffing on top.

Seal pot with air fryer lid and select bake mode then set the temperature to 350° F and timer for 40 minutes.

Serve and enjoy.

Nutrition:

Calories 317, Fat 10.8g, Carbohydrates 17.7g, Sugar 3g, Protein 35.1g, Cholesterol 88mg.

233. Spinach risotto

Preparation time: 10 minutes | Cooking Time: 10 minutes | Servings: 4

Ingredients:

1 1/2 cups arborio rice

8 oz mushrooms, sliced

1 1/2 cups butternut squash, peeled and diced

1/2 cup dry white wine

3 1/2 cups vegetable broth

1 bell pepper, diced

1 tbsp garlic, minced

1 onion, chopped

3 cups spinach, chopped

1/4 tsp oregano

1/2 tsp coriander

1 tbsp olive oil

1 tsp pepper

1 tsp salt

Directions:

Add oil into the inner pot of Pressure Pot duo crisp and set pot on sauté mode.

Add squash, bell pepper, garlic, and onion and sauté for 5 minutes.

Add remaining ingredients except for spinach and stir well.

Seal the pot with a pressure-cooking lid and cook on high for 5 minutes.

Once done, release pressure using a quick release. Remove lid.

Add spinach and stir well and let it sit for 5 minutes.

Stir well and serve.

Nutrition:

Calories 411, Fat 5.5g, Carbohydrates 73g, Sugar 5.8g, Protein 12.7g, Cholesterol 0mg.

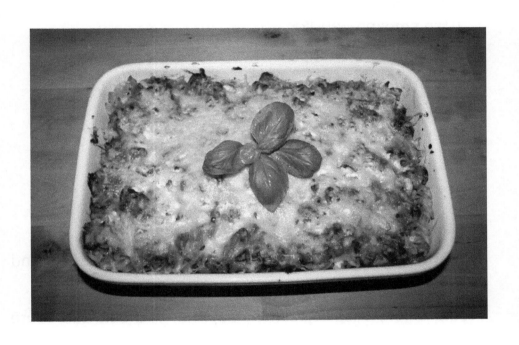

Chickpea Stew

Preparation time: 10 minutes | Cooking Time: 25 minutes | Servings: 6

Ingredients:

28 oz cans chickpeas, rinsed and drained

1/2 tsp ground cumin

1 tsp smoked paprika

2 large onion, chopped

2 tbsp olive oil

24 oz can tomato

1/4 cup dates, pitted and chopped

1/4 tsp allspice

1/2 tsp sea salt

Directions:

Add oil into the inner pot of Pressure Pot duo crisp and set pot on sauté mode.

Add onion, allspice, cumin, paprika, and salt and sauté for 5 minutes.

Add remaining ingredients and stir well.

Seal the pot with a pressure-cooking lid and cook on high for 20 minutes.

Once done, allow to release pressure naturally. Remove lid.

Stir and serve.

Nutrition:

Calories 264, Fat 6.4g, Carbohydrates 46.2g, Sugar 10.7g, Protein 8.4g, Cholesterol 0mg.

Quick Veggie Pasta

Preparation time: 10 minutes | Cooking Time: 4 minutes | Servings: 4

Ingredients:

1/2 lb pasta, uncooked

1/4 green onion, sliced

1/4 tsp red chili flakes

1 tsp ground ginger

1 tbsp garlic, minced

3 tbsp coconut amino

2 cups vegetable broth

1 1/2 cups baby spinach, chopped

1 cup frozen peas

8 oz mushrooms, sliced

2 carrots, peeled and chopped

1/4 tsp pepper

1 tsp salt

Directions:

Add all ingredients except spinach into the inner pot of Pressure Pot duo crisp and stir well.

Seal the pot with a pressure-cooking lid and cook on high for 4 minutes.

Once done, allow to release pressure naturally. Remove lid.

Add spinach and stir well and let it sit for 5 minutes.

Serve and enjoy.

Nutrition:

Calories 258, Fat 2.3g, Carbohydrates 45.9g, Sugar 4.8g, Protein 13.4g, Cholesterol 41mg.

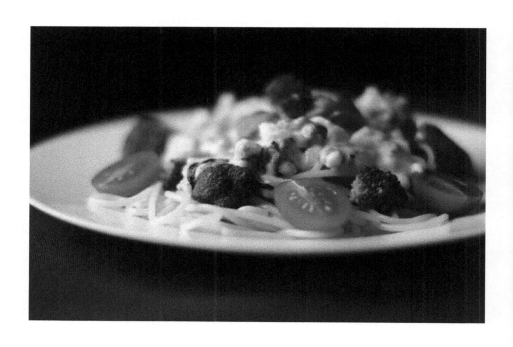

Baked Beans

Preparation time: 10 minutes | Cooking Time: 40 minutes | Servings: 4

Ingredients:

1 cup navy beans, dry, soaked overnight, and drained

2 tbsp tomato paste

1/2 tbsp vinegar

1/2 tbsp Worcestershire sauce

1/2 tsp mustard

1 onion, chopped

1 tbsp olive oil

1/2 cup water

1/2 cup vegetable stock

1 1/2 tbsp molasses

2 tbsp brown sugar

1/2 tsp pepper

1/2 tsp sea salt

Directions:

Add oil into the inner pot of Pressure Pot duo crisp and set pot on sauté mode.

Add onion and sauté for 3 minutes.

Add remaining ingredients and stir to combine.

Seal the pot with a pressure-cooking lid and cook on high for 40 minutes.

Once done, release pressure using a quick release. Remove lid.

Stir well and serve.

Nutrition:

Calories 267, Fat 4.5g, Carbohydrates 46.5g, Sugar 13.2g, Protein 12.5g, Cholesterol 0mg.

Easy Lentil Tacos

Preparation time: 10 minutes | Cooking Time: 15 minutes | Servings: 4

Ingredients:

2 cups brown lentils

1 tsp chili powder

1/2 tsp onion powder

1/2 cup tomato paste

4 cups vegetable broth

1/2 tsp ground cumin

1/2 tsp garlic powder

1 tsp salt

Directions:

Add all ingredients into the inner pot of Pressure Pot duo crisp and stir well.

Seal the pot with a pressure-cooking lid and cook on high for 15 minutes.

Once done, release pressure using a quick release. Remove lid.

Stir well and serve.

Nutrition:

Calories 108, Fat 1.9g, Carbohydrates 13g, Sugar 5.5g, Protein 9g, Cholesterol 0mg.

Rice Black Bean Burritos

Preparation time: 10 minutes | Cooking Time: 24 minutes | Servings: 4

Ingredients:

1 cup black beans, dry, soaked overnight, and drained

2 cups brown rice

1 tsp paprika

1 tbsp ground cumin

1 onion, chopped

1 tbsp chili powder

4 1/2 vegetable broth

1 cup tomato puree

1 tsp olive oil

1 tsp garlic, minced

Directions:

Add oil into the inner pot of Pressure Pot duo crisp and set pot on sauté mode.

Add garlic and onion and sauté for 2 minutes.

Add 2 cups of broth and rice. Stir well.

Seal the pot with a pressure-cooking lid and cook on high for 12 minutes.

Once done, release pressure using a quick release. Remove lid.

Add beans, remaining broth, chili powder, cumin, tomato puree, and paprika. Stir well.

Seal the pot again with a pressure-cooking lid and cook on high for 10 minutes.

Once done, allow to release pressure naturally. Remove lid.

Serve in a tortilla.

Nutrition:

Calories 618, Fat 5.3g, Carbohydrates 124.3g, Sugar 5.5g, Protein 20.7g, Cholesterol 0mg.

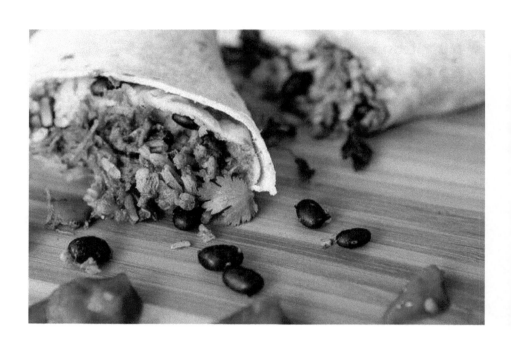

Veggie Risotto

Preparation time: 10 minutes | Cooking Time: 13 minutes | Servings: 4

Ingredients:

1 cup arborio rice

1/2 cup peas

1 red pepper, diced

1 onion, chopped

1 tsp dried mix herbs

3 cups vegetable stock

1 tbsp olive oil

1 tsp garlic, minced

1/2 cup corn

1/4 pepper

1/2 tsp salt

Directions:

Add oil into the inner pot of Pressure Pot duo crisp and set pot on sauté mode.

Add onion and garlic and sauté for 5 minutes.

Add rice and stir well. Add remaining ingredients and stir well.

Seal the pot with a pressure-cooking lid and cook on high for 8 minutes.

Once done, release pressure using a quick release. Remove lid.

Stir and serve.

Nutrition:

Calories 288, Fat 4.2g, Carbohydrates 56g, Sugar 5.4g, Protein 6.7g, Cholesterol 0mg.

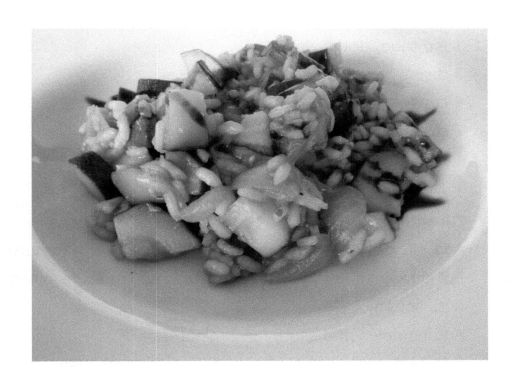

Tasty Pumpkin Risotto

Preparation time: 10 minutes | Cooking Time: 15 minutes | Servings: 8

Ingredients:

3 cups pumpkin, diced

1 cup cream cheese

1 tsp sage, dried

3 tbsp olive oil

4 cups vegetable broth

2 tbsp white wine

1 onion, chopped

1 tsp garlic, minced

Directions:

Add oil, garlic, and onion into the inner pot of Pressure Pot duo crisp and set pot on sauté mode. Sauté onion until soften.

Add pumpkin and sauté for a minute.

Add white wine, sage, rice, and broth and stir well.

Seal the pot with a pressure-cooking lid and cook on high for 10 minutes.

Once done, allow to release pressure naturally. Remove lid.

Add cream cheese and stir well.

Serve and enjoy.

Nutrition:

Calories 377, Fat 16.6g, Carbohydrates 48g, Sugar 4.1g, Protein 9g, Cholesterol 32mg.

Spicy Chicken Wings

Preparation Time: 10 minutes | Cooking Time: 20 minutes | Servings: 4

Ingredients:

2 lbs frozen chicken wings

2 tbsp apple cider vinegar

2 tbsp butter, melted

1/2 cup hot pepper sauce

1/2 cup water

1/2 tsp paprika

1 oz ranch seasoning

Directions:

Add water, vinegar, butter, and hot pepper sauce into the Pressure Pot duo crisp.

Add chicken wings and stir well.

Seal the pot with a pressure-cooking lid and cook on high for 5 minutes.

Once done, release pressure using a quick release. Remove lid.

Sprinkle paprika and ranch seasoning over the chicken.

Seal the pot with an air fryer lid and select air fry mode and cook at 375° F for 15 minutes.

Toss wings in sauce and serve.

Nutrition:

Calories 521, Fat 38.2g, Carbohydrates 0.2g, Sugar 0.1g, Protein 36.6g, Cholesterol 167mg.

Cheesy Chicken Wings

Preparation Time: 10 minutes | Cooking Time: 18 minutes | Servings: 4

Ingredients:

2 lbs chicken wings

1/2 cup chicken stock

1 tsp season salt

For sauce:

1/2 cup parmesan cheese, grated

1 tbsp garlic, crushed

1 stick butter, melted

1/2 tsp black pepper

1/2 tsp dried parsley flakes

1 tsp garlic powder

Directions:

Season chicken wings with seasoned salt.

Add chicken wings to the inner pot of Pressure Pot duo crisp along with the chicken stock.

Seal the pot with a pressure-cooking lid and cook on high for 8 minutes.

Meanwhile, mix butter, pepper, parmesan cheese, parsley flakes, garlic powder, and garlic. Set aside.

Once chicken wings are done then release pressures using a quick release. Remove lid.

Remove chicken wings from the pot and clean the pot.

Spray Pressure Pot air fryer basket with cooking spray and place in the pot.

Toss chicken wings with melted butter and add them into the air fryer basket.

Seal the pot with an air fryer lid and select broil mode and cook for 10 minutes.

Serve and enjoy.

Nutrition:

Calories 652, Fat 40.6g, Carbohydrates 1.6g, Sugar 0.3g, Protein 67.3g, Cholesterol 265mg.

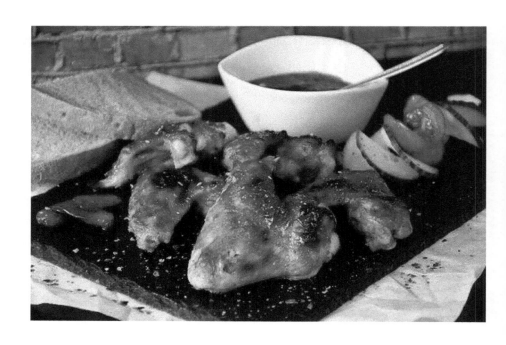

Chicken Rice

Preparation Time: 10 minutes | Cooking Time: 12 minutes | Servings: 6

Ingredients:

2 lbs chicken thighs, skinless, boneless, and cut into pieces

18 oz enchilada sauce

15 oz frozen mixed vegetables

1 oz taco seasoning

2 cups rice, uncooked

1 cup chicken stock

Directions:

Spray Pressure Pot duo crisp inner pot with cooking spray and set the pot on sauté mode.

Season chicken with taco seasoning and place in the pot.

Sear chicken until brown from all the sides, about 10 minutes.

Add rice, stock, enchilada sauce, and vegetables and stir well.

Seal the pot with a pressure-cooking lid and cook on high for 2 minutes.

Once done, allow to release pressure naturally for 10 minutes then release remaining pressure using a quick release. Remove lid.

Stir well and serve.

Nutrition:

Calories 787, Fat 15.2g, Carbohydrates 114.6g, Sugar 2.9g, Protein 60.2g, Cholesterol 136mg.

Spicy Chicken Breast

Preparation Time: 10 minutes | Cooking Time: 35 minutes | Servings: 2

Ingredients:

2 chicken breasts, bone-in, and skin-on

1 tbsp ground fennel

1 tbsp chili powder

1 tbsp olive oil

1 tsp ground cumin

1 tsp garlic powder

1 tsp onion powder

1 tbsp paprika

1/2 tsp black pepper

1 tsp sea salt

Directions:

In a small bowl, mix all dried spices.

Brush chicken with olive oil and rub with spice mixture.

Place chicken in the Pressure Pot air fryer basket and place basket in the pot.

Seal the pot with an air fryer lid and select air fry mode and cook at 375° F for 35 minutes.

Serve and enjoy.

Nutrition:

Calories 108, Fat 8.9g, Carbohydrates 8.3g, Sugar 1.4g, Protein 2.3g, Cholesterol 1mg.

Tasty Butter Chicken

Preparation Time: 10 minutes | Cooking Time: 8 minutes | Servings: 6

Ingredients:

3 lbs chicken breasts, boneless, skinless, and cut into cubes

1/2 cup butter, cut into cubes

2 tbsp tomato paste

1 tsp turmeric powder

2 tbsp garam masala

1 tbsp ginger paste

1 tbsp garlic paste

1 onion, diced

1/4 cup fresh cilantro, chopped

1/2 cup heavy cream

1 1/4 cup tomato sauce

2/3 cup chicken stock

1 1/2 tsp olive oil

1 tsp kosher salt

Directions:

Add 3 tbsp butter and oil in the inner pot of Pressure Pot duo crisp and set pot on sauté mode.

Add garlic paste and onion and sauté for a minute.

Add chicken, tomato sauce, stock, tomato paste, turmeric, garam masala, ginger paste, and salt and stir to combine.

Seal the pot with a pressure-cooking lid and cook on high for 5 minutes.

Once done, release pressure using a quick release. Remove lid.

Set pot on sauté mode. Add remaining butter and heavy cream and cook for 2 minutes.

Stir well and serve.

Nutrition:

Calories 643, Fat 37.3g, Carbohydrates 7.2g, Sugar 3.8g, Protein 67.4g, Cholesterol 256mg.

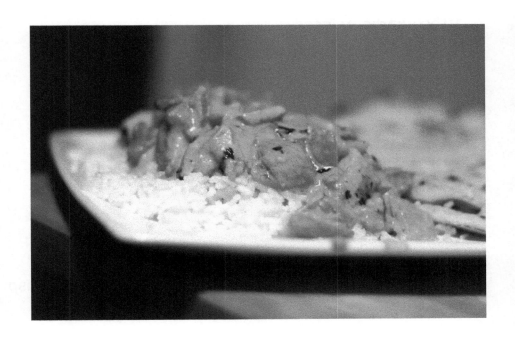

Chicken Pasta

Preparation Time: 10 minutes | Cooking Time: 15 minutes | Servings: 4

Ingredients:

1 lb chicken breasts, boneless and skinless, cut into bite-size pieces

1 tbsp garlic, minced

2 bell peppers, seeded and diced

2 tbsp olive oil

1 onion, diced

1 cup chicken stock

3 tbsp fajita seasoning

8 oz penne pasta, dry

7 oz can tomato

Directions:

Add olive oil in the inner pot of Pressure Pot duo crisp and set pot on sauté mode.

Add chicken and half fajita seasoning in the pot and sauté chicken for 3-5 minutes.

Add garlic, bell pepper, onions, and remaining fajitas seasoning and sauté for 2 minutes.

Add tomatoes, stock, and pasta and stir well.

Seal the pot with a pressure-cooking lid and cook on high for 6 minutes.

Once done, release pressure using a quick release. Remove lid.

Set pot on sauté mode and cook for 1-2 minutes.

Serve and enjoy.

Nutrition:

Calories 509, Fat 17g, Carbohydrates 46.2g, Sugar 6.1g, Protein 40.9g, Cholesterol 142mg.

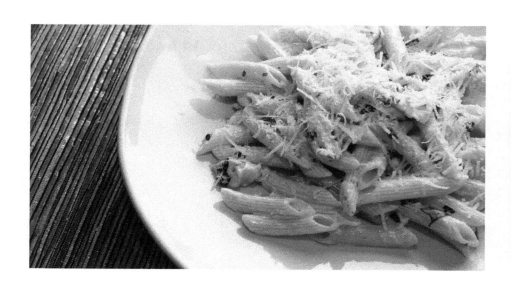

Easy Cheesy Chicken

Preparation Time: 10 minutes | Cooking Time: 17 minutes | Servings: 6

Ingredients:

1 1/2 lbs chicken tenders

25 oz tomato sauce

2 tbsp butter

1/2 cup olive oil

1/2 tsp garlic powder

1/2 cup parmesan cheese, grated

2 cups mozzarella cheese, shredded

Directions:

Add olive oil into the inner pot of Pressure Pot duo crisp and set pot on sauté mode.

Add chicken and sauté until lightly brown from both the sides.

Add garlic powder, tomato sauce, butter, and parmesan cheese on top of the chicken.

Seal the pot with a pressure-cooking lid and cook on high for 15 minutes.

Once done, release pressure using a quick release. Remove lid.

Sprinkle mozzarella cheese on top of chicken. Cover pot with air fryer lid and select broil mode and cook for 1-2 minutes.

Serve and enjoy.

Nutrition:

Calories 457, Fat 31.4g, Carbohydrates 6.9g, Sugar 5.1g, Protein 37.9g, Cholesterol 118mg.

Creamy Italian Chicken

Preparation Time: 10 minutes | Cooking Time: 10 minutes | Servings: 8

Ingredients:

2 lbs chicken breasts, skinless and boneless

1 cup chicken stock

1/4 cup butter

14 oz can cream of chicken soup

8 oz cream cheese

1 tbsp Italian seasoning

Directions:

Add the chicken stock into the inner pot of Pressure Pot duo crisp.

Add cream of chicken soup, Italian seasoning, and butter into the pot and stir well.

Seal the pot with a pressure-cooking lid and cook on high for 10 minutes.

Once done, release pressure using a quick release. Remove lid.

Add cream cheese and stir until cheese is melted

Serve and enjoy.

Nutrition:

Calories 416, Fat 27.5g, Carbohydrates 4.6g, Sugar 0.6g, Protein 36.3g, Cholesterol 153mg.

Paprika Chicken

Preparation Time: 10 minutes | Cooking Time: 30 minutes | Servings: 4

Ingredients:

4 chicken breasts, skinless and boneless, cut into chunks

2 tsp garlic, minced

2 tbsp smoked paprika

3 tbsp olive oil

2 tbsp lemon juice

Pepper

Salt

Directions:

In a small bowl, mix garlic, lemon juice, paprika, oil, pepper, and salt.

Rub chicken with garlic mixture.

Add chicken into the Pressure Pot air fryer basket and place basket in the pot.

Seal the pot with an air fryer lid and select bake mode and cook at 350° F for 30 minutes.

Serve and enjoy.

Nutrition:

Calories 381, Fat 21.8g, Carbohydrates 2.6g, Sugar 0.5g, Protein 42.9g, Cholesterol 130mg.

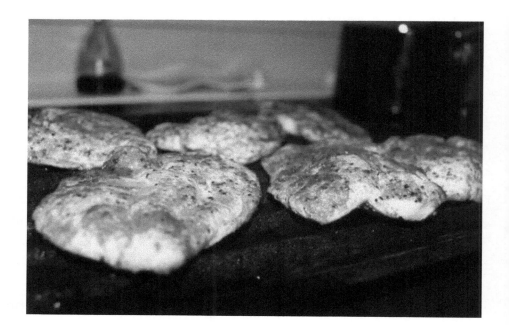

Garlic Lemon Chicken

Preparation Time: 10 minutes | Cooking Time: 40 minutes | Servings: 4

Ingredients:

2 lbs chicken drumsticks

4 tbsp butter

2 tbsp parsley, chopped

1 fresh lemon juice

10 garlic cloves, minced

2 tbsp olive oil

Pepper

Salt

Directions:

Add butter, parsley, lemon juice, garlic, oil, pepper, and salt into the mixing bowl and mix well.

Add chicken to the bowl and toss until well coated.

Transfer chicken into the Pressure Pot air fryer basket and place basket in the pot.

Seal the pot with an air fryer lid and select bake mode and cook at 400° F for 40 minutes.

Serve and enjoy.

Nutrition:

Calories 560, Fat 31.6g, Carbohydrates 2.9g, Sugar 0.4g, Protein 63.1g, Cholesterol 230mg.

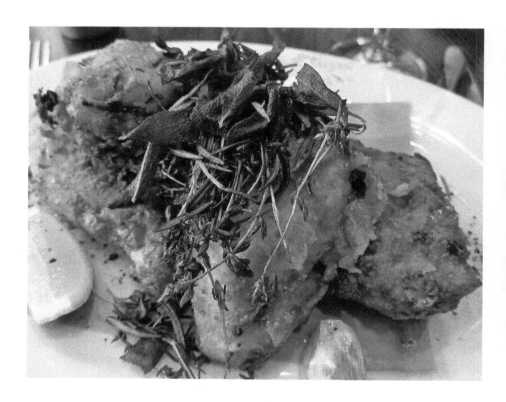

Flavorful Herb Chicken

Preparation Time: 10 minutes | Cooking Time: 4 hours |
Servings: 6

Ingredients:

6 chicken breasts, skinless and boneless

1 onion, sliced

14 oz can tomato, diced

1 tsp dried basil

1 tsp dried rosemary

1 tbsp olive oil

1/2 cup balsamic vinegar

1/2 tsp thyme

1 tsp dried oregano

4 garlic cloves

Pepper

Salt

Directions:

Add all ingredients into the inner pot of Pressure Pot
duo crisp and stir well.

Seal the pot with a pressure-cooking lid and select slow
cook mode and cook on high for 4 hours.

Stir well and serve.

Nutrition:

Calories 328, Fat 13.3g, Carbohydrates 6.3g, Sugar 3.1g, Protein 43.2g, Cholesterol 130mg.

Chicken Fajitas

Preparation Time: 10 minutes | Cooking Time: 10 minutes | Servings: 6

Ingredients:

4 chicken breasts, skinless and boneless

1/2 cup bell pepper, sliced

1/2 cup water

1 packet fajita seasoning

1 onion, sliced

1/4 tsp garlic powder

Directions:

Add all ingredients into the inner pot of Pressure Pot duo crisp and stir well.

Seal the pot with a pressure-cooking lid and cook on high for 10 minutes.

Once done, release pressure using a quick release. Remove lid.

Shred chicken using a fork and stir well.

Serve and enjoy.

Nutrition:

Calories 198, Fat 7.3g, Carbohydrates 3.1g, Sugar 1.3g, Protein 28.5g, Cholesterol 87mg.

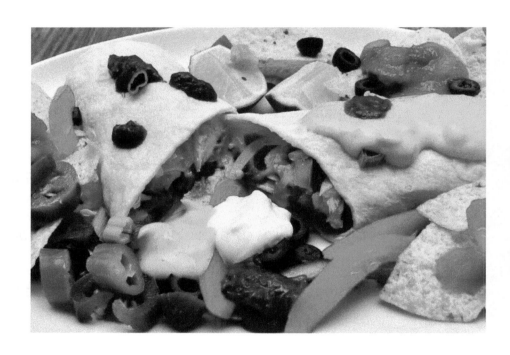

Jamaican Chicken

Preparation Time: 10 minutes | Cooking Time: 15 minutes | Servings: 6

Ingredients:

6 chicken drumsticks

1 tbsp jerk seasoning

3 tbsp soy sauce

1/4 cup red wine vinegar

1/4 cup brown sugar

1/2 cup ketchup

1 tsp salt

Directions:

Add all ingredients except chicken into the inner pot of Pressure Pot duo crisp and stir well.

Add chicken and stir to coat.

Seal the pot with a pressure-cooking lid and cook on high for 10 minutes.

Once done, release pressure using a quick release. Remove lid.

Remove chicken from pot. Set pot on sauté mode and cook sauce for 5 minutes.

Pour sauce over chicken and serve.

Nutrition:

Calories 126, Fat 2.7g, Carbohydrates 11.7g, Sugar 10.6g, Protein 13.5g, Cholesterol 40mg.

Flavorful Lemon Chicken

Preparation Time: 10 minutes | Cooking Time: 4 hours 5 minutes | Servings: 4

Ingredients:

20 oz chicken breasts, skinless, boneless, and cut into pieces

1 tsp dried parsley

2 tbsp olive oil

2 tbsp butter

3 tbsp flour

1/4 cup chicken broth

1/2 cup fresh lemon juice

1/8 tsp dried thyme Fla

1/4 tsp dried basil

1/2 tsp dried oregano

1 tsp salt

Directions:

In a bowl, toss chicken with flour.

Heat butter and oil in a pan over medium-high heat.

Add chicken to the pan and sear until brown.

Transfer chicken into the inner pot of Pressure Pot duo crisp.

Add remaining ingredients on top of chicken.

Seal the pot with a pressure-cooking lid and select slow cook mode and cook on low for 4 hours.

Serve and enjoy.

Nutrition:

Calories 412, Fat 23.7g, Carbohydrates 5.3g, Sugar 0.7g, Protein 42.3g, Cholesterol 141mg.

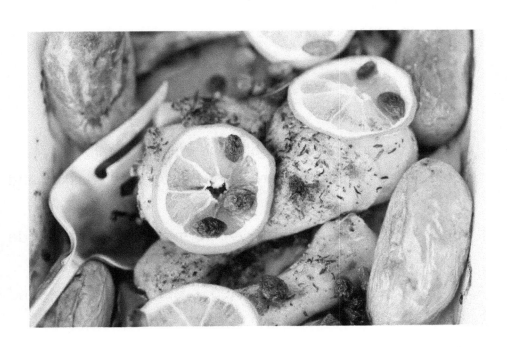

Roasted Broccoli with Cashews

Preparation time: 10 minutes | Cooking Time: 15 minutes | Servings: 2

Ingredients:

3 cups broccoli florets

1/2 tbsp coconut amino

1/4 cup cashews, roasted

1 tbsp olive oil

1/2 tsp salt

Directions:

In a bowl, add broccoli, salt, and oil. Toss well.

Place broccoli into the Pressure Pot air fryer basket and place the basket into the pot.

Seal the pot with an air fryer lid and select bake mode and cook at 375° F for 15 minutes.

In a large bowl, add roasted broccoli, cashews, and coconut amino and toss well.

Serve and enjoy.

Nutrition:

Calories 209, Fat 15.4g, Carbohydrates 15.4g, Sugar 3.2g, Protein 6.4g, Cholesterol 0mg.

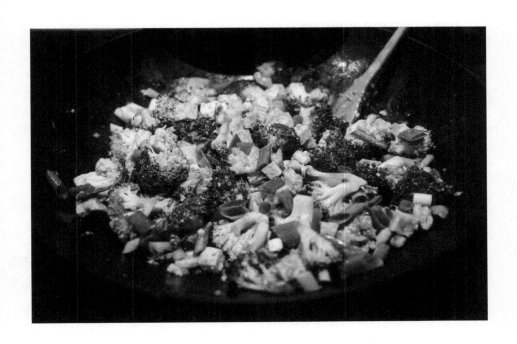

Crispy Air-Fried Brussels Sprouts

Preparation time: 5 minutes | Cooking Time: 16 minutes | Servings: 2

Ingredients:

2 tbsp. Parmesan (freshly grated

1/2 lb. Of brussels sprouts (thinly sliced

1 tsp. Garlic powder

1 tbsp. Extra-virgin olive oil

Caesar dressing for dipping

Black pepper (freshly ground

Kosher salt

Directions:

Add oil, brussels sprouts, garlic powder, and parmesan in a large mixing bowl.

Toss to combine thoroughly. Season with salt and pepper.

Put coated sprouts in the air fryer basket.

Insert trivet into your Pressure Pot and lay the air fryer basket on top.

Attach the air fryer lid and cook at 350° F for 8 minutes.

Toss and cook for another 8 minutes until sprouts are crisp and golden brown.

Garnish with parmesan. You may serve it with Caesar salad for a dip.

Nutrition:

Calories 02, Carbohydrates 15.9g, Fat 12.32g, Protein 6.89g, Sugar 4.18g, Sodium 330mg.

Pressure Pot Air-Fried Green Beans

Preparation time: 5 minutes | Cooking Time: 15 minutes | Servings: 4

Ingredients:

1 tbsp. Olive oil or cooking spray

1 lb. Fresh green beans (with ends trimmed and cut into halves

1/2 tsp. Garlic powder

Salt and pepper to taste

Fresh lemon slices

Directions

Combine green beans with garlic powder in a bowl and season with salt and pepper.

Arrange seasoned green beans in the air fryer basket

Place the basket inside the Pressure Pot air fryer crisp and attach the air fryer lid.

Make sure it locks before setting it to air frying mode. Cook at 360° F for 10-14 minutes.

Toss and shake two times while cooking.

Adjust seasoning to taste if needed serve garnished with lemon slices.

Nutrition:

Calories 82, Fat 5.66g, Carbohydrates 6.3g, Protein 1.5 g, Sugar 1.7g, Fiber 2.4g, Sodium 46mg.

Roasted Asparagus in Pressure Pot Air Fryer

Preparation time: 4 minutes | Cooking Time: 10 minutes | Servings: 4

Ingredients:

1 lb. Asparagus with ends trimmed

1-2 tsp. Olive oil

Salt and black pepper to taste

Directions:

Place pieces of asparagus in a shallow dish and coat them with olive oil.

Season it with salt and pepper.

Make sure to properly coat asparagus ends to prevent them from burning or drying out quickly.

Place asparagus inside the air fryer basket and put it inside Pressure Pot air fryer crisp.

Choose the air fryer lift for cover, secure, and set to air frying at 380° F for 7-10 minutes.

Shake basket halfway through cooking to cook asparagus evenly.

Taste for seasoning and tenderness.

Adjust if needed.

Serve warm.

Nutrition:

Calories 52kcal, Fat 1.97g, Carbohydrates 5.72g, Protein 2.95g, Sugar 2.4g, Fiber 2.4g, Sodium 273mg.

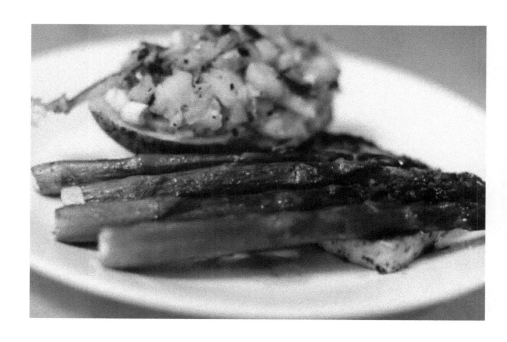

Air Fryer Crispy Broccoli

Preparation time: 5 minutes | Cooking Time: 10 minutes | Servings: 4

Ingredients:

2 tbsp. Cooking oil

1 lb. Broccoli (cut into bite-size pieces

½ tsp. Garlic powder

Salt and pepper to taste

Fresh lemon wedges

Directions

Add broccoli to a large bowl and drizzle evenly with olive oil.

Season broccoli with garlic powder, salt, and pepper.

Put in an Pressure Pot air fryer crisp air fryer basket and cover with the air fryer lid.

Air fry 380° F for 12-15 minutes, flipping and shaking 3 times through cooking or cook until crispy.

Serve with lemon wedges.

Nutrition:

Calories 104 kcal, Fat 7.41g, Carbohydrates 5.42 g, Protein 3.93g, Sugar 1.32g, Fiber 3.3g, Sodium 39mg.

Air Fried Acorn Squash

Preparation time: 15 minutes | Cooking Time: 20 minutes | Servings: 4

Ingredients:

1 acorn squash

3 tbsp. Butter (melted

2 tsp. Brown sugar

1/2 tsp. Kosher salt

Black pepper to taste

Optional toppings: melted butter, roasted nuts (chopped), pomegranate seeds

Direction:

Cleanse squash and trim ends. Cut in half and core to remove seeds. Cut into about half an inch thick.

Combine in a bowl brown sugar, melted butter. Season with salt and pepper.

Add in the acorn squash and toss to coat.

Place coated squash into the air fryer basket and attach the air fryer lid to the Pressure Pot. Set to air fry at 375° F for 15-20 minutes or until tender, flipping after 10 minutes of cooking.

Once done, serve in a platter drizzled with melted butter, pomegranate seeds, and chopped nuts. Taste for seasoning and adjust flavor if needed.

Nutrition:

Calories 152g, Fat 7.73g, Carbohydrates 27.74g, Protein 2.63g, Sugar 12.45g, Fiber 4.6g, Sodium 352mg.

Pressure Pot Air-Fried Avocado

Preparation time: 10 minutes | Cooking Time: 10 minutes | Servings: 2

Ingredients:

1/2 cup all-purpose flour

2 avocados

2 large eggs

2 tbsp. Canola mayonnaise

1 tbsp. Apple cider vinegar

1 tbsp. Sriracha chili sauce

1 1/2 tsp. Black pepper

1/4 tsp. Kosher salt

1/2 cup panko breadcrumbs

1/4 cup no-salt-added ketchup

1 tbsp. Water

Cooking spray

Directions:

Cut avocado into 4 wedges each. Prepare 3 shallow dishes.

In the first shallow dish, combine avocado wedges with flour and pepper.

In another dish, lightly beat eggs

Place breadcrumbs in the third dish

First, dredge avocado wedges in the flour mixture, one after the other. After coating with flour, shake lightly to remove excess flour and dip the avocado to the egg mixture, likewise shaking lightly to drip off excess liquid. Finally, dip each wedge to the breadcrumbs coating them evenly on all sides, and spray with cooking oil.

Arrange avocado wedged in the Pressure Pot duo air fryer basket, place it inside the pot, and cover it with the air fryer lid. Set to air fry at 400° F until wedges turn golden brown, turning them over halfway through cooking. Remove avocado wedges from the fryer and sprinkle them with salt.

Meanwhile, while waiting for the avocado wedges to get cooked, mix mayonnaise, ketchup, apple cider vinegar, and sriracha sauce in a small bowl.

Serve the prepared sauce with the avocado wedges while still warm.

Nutrition:

Calories 274, Fat 18g, Carbohydrates 23g, Protein 5g, Sugar 5g, Fiber 7g, Sodium 306mg.

Mediterranean Veggies in Pressure Pot Air Fryer

Preparation time: 5 minutes | Cooking Time: 20 minutes | Servings: 4

Ingredients:

1 1 large courgetti

50 g cherry tomatoes

1 green pepper

1 medium carrot

1 large parsnip

1 tsp. Mixed herbs

2 tbsp. Honey

Tbsp. Olive oil

2 tsp. Garlic puree

1 tsp. Mustard

Salt and pepper to taste

Directions:

Slice up the courgetti and the green pepper.

Peel and dice the carrots and the parsnips

Add them all altogether in the air fryer basket of the Pressure Pot duo along with raw cherry tomatoes. Drizzle with three tablespoons of olive oil.

Place the air fryer in the pot and air fry for 15 minutes at 356° F using an Pressure Pot air fryer crisp air fryer. Sprinkle with more salt if needed and serve.

Nutrition:

Calories 281, Fat 21g, Carbohydrates 21g, Protein 2g, Sugar 13g, Fiber 3g, Sodium 36mg.

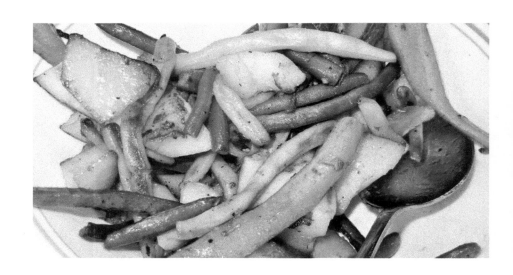

Lightning Source UK Ltd.
Milton Keynes UK
UKHW020809180621
385732UK00001B/34